Heart

appuccio

LONDON

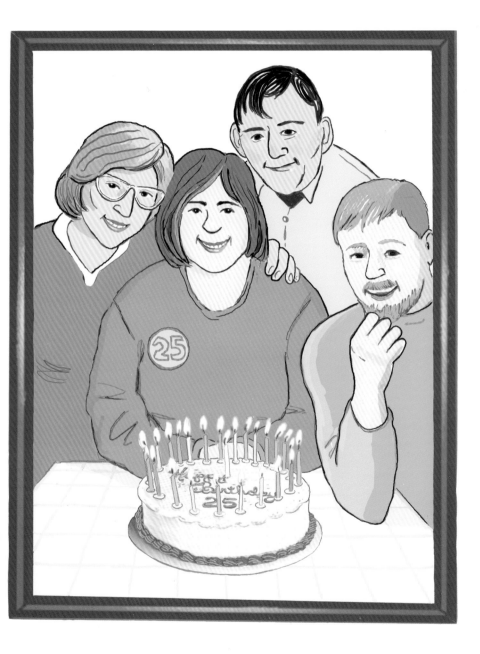

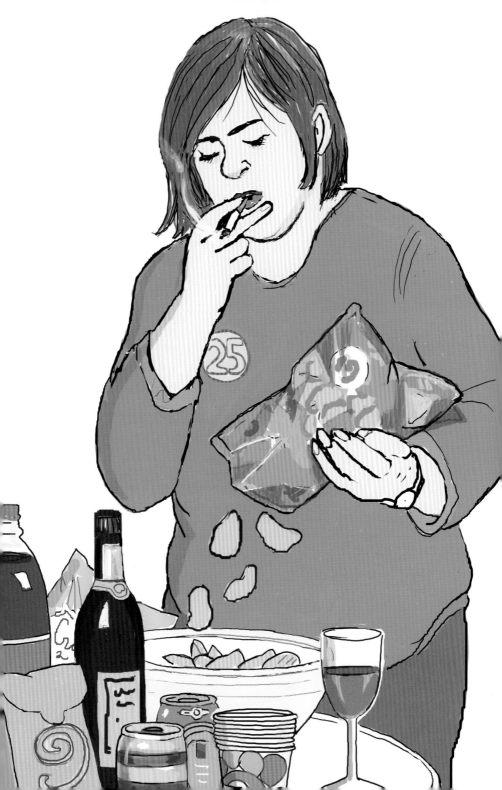

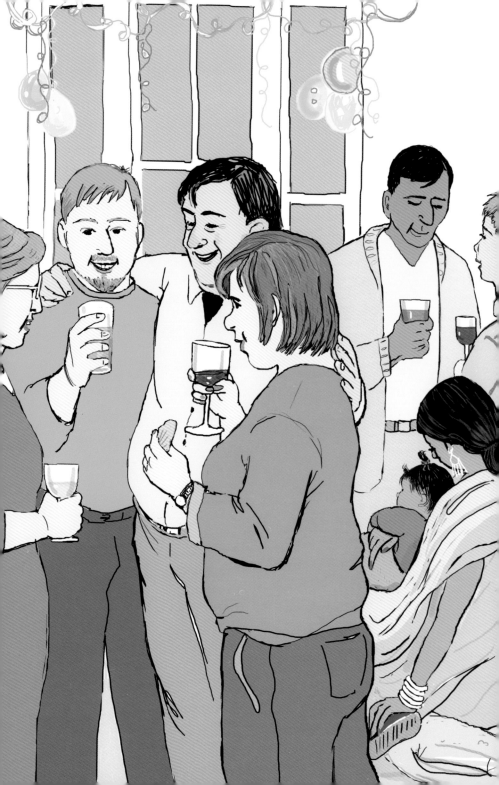

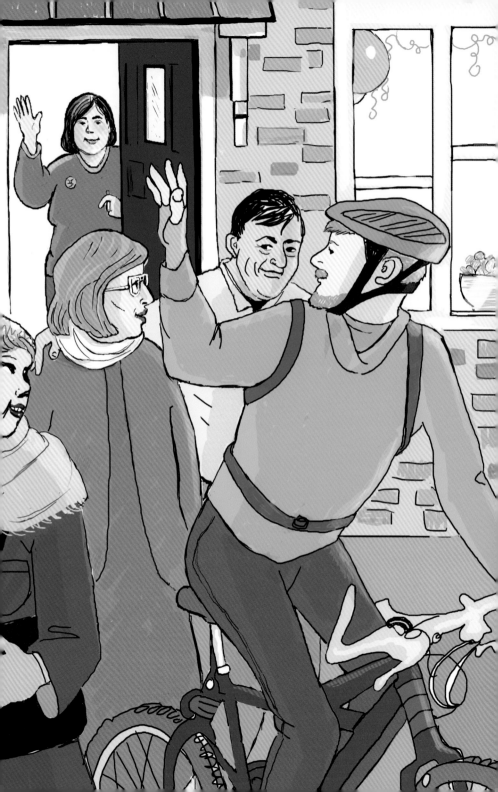

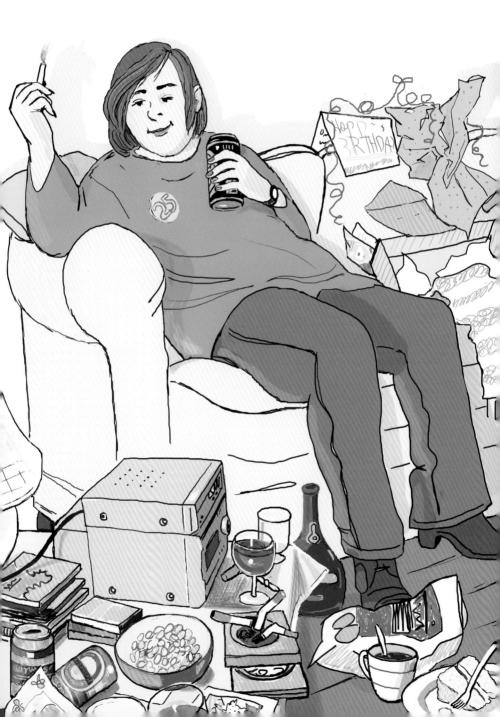

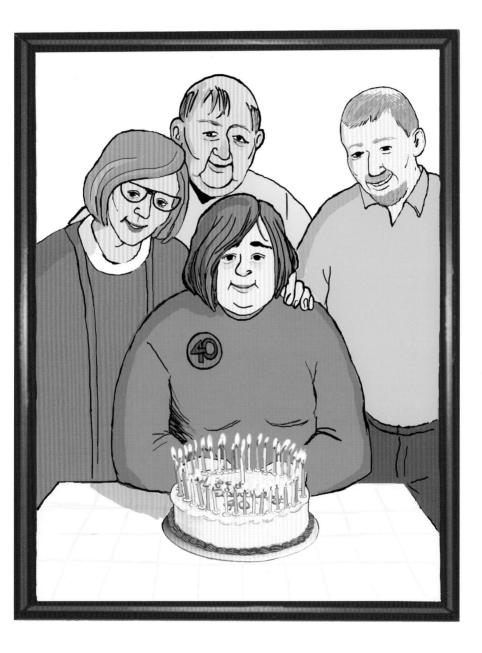

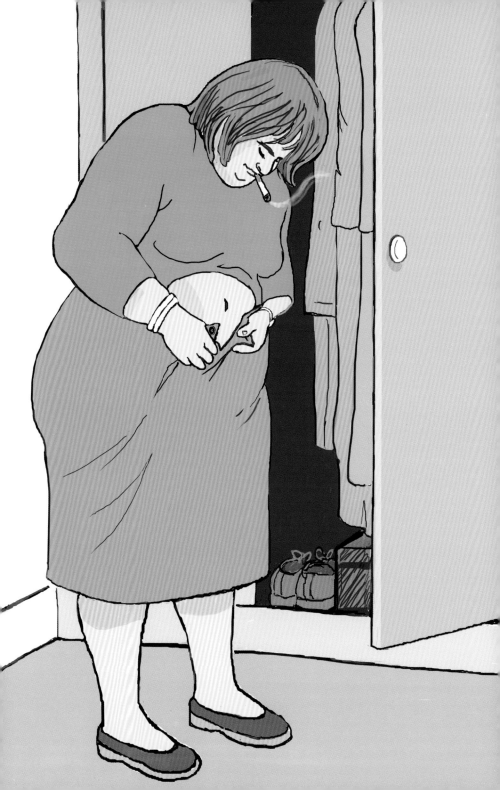

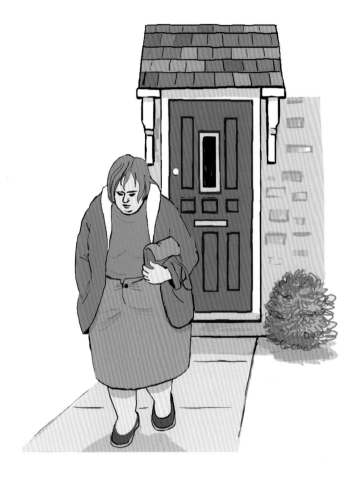

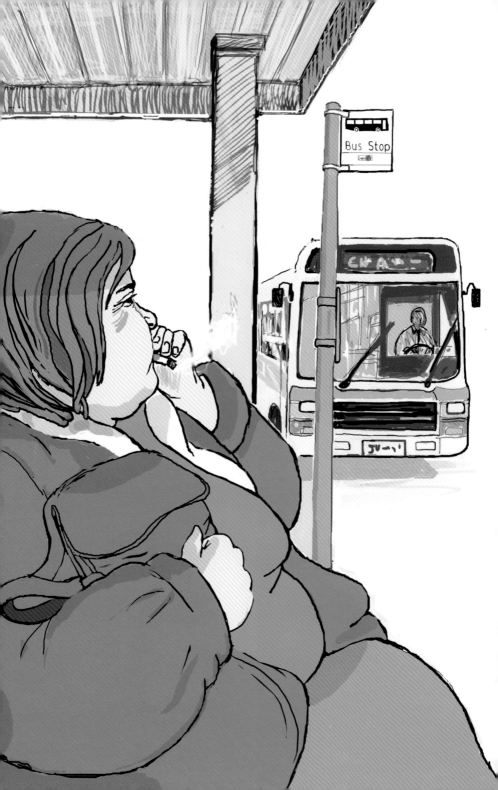

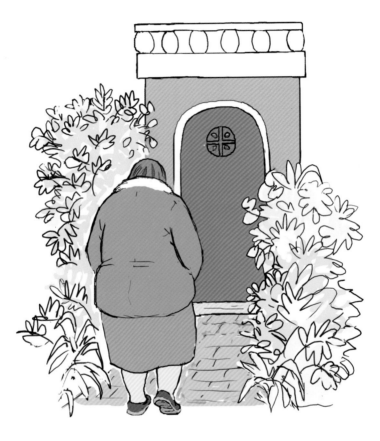

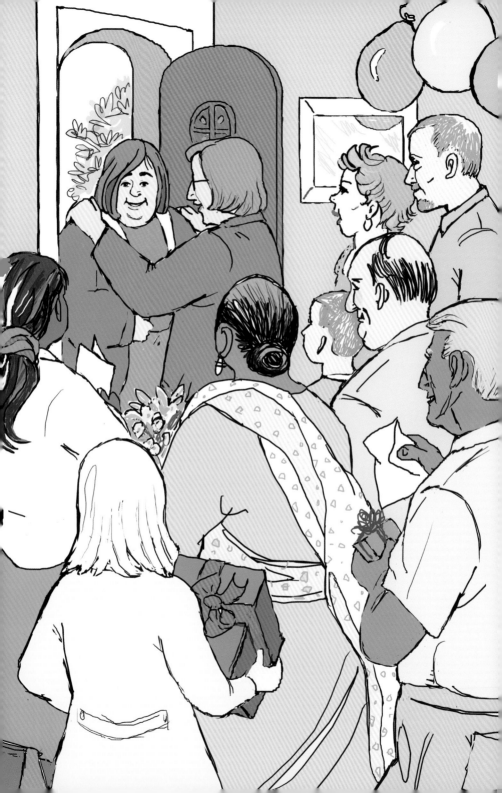

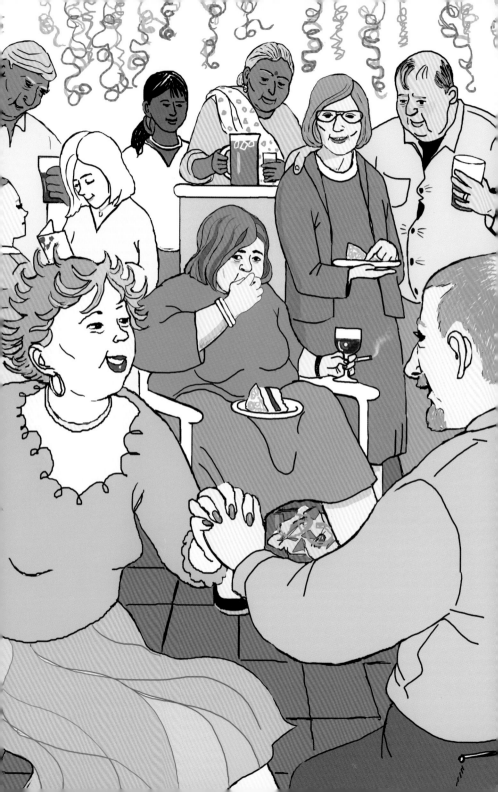

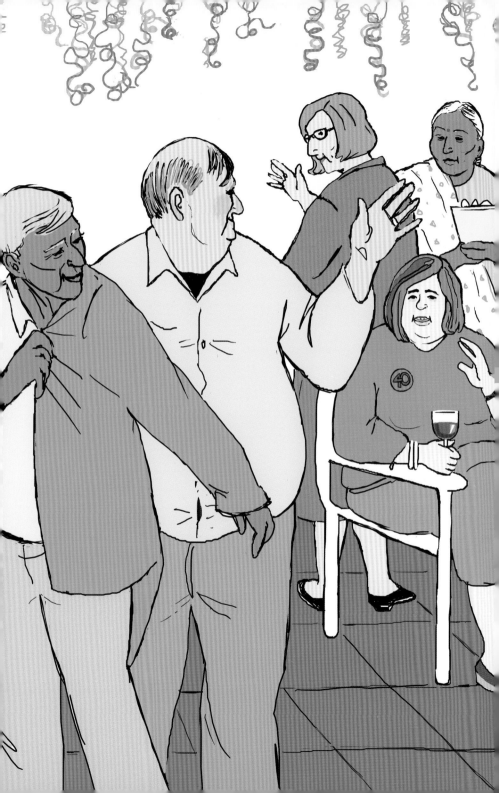

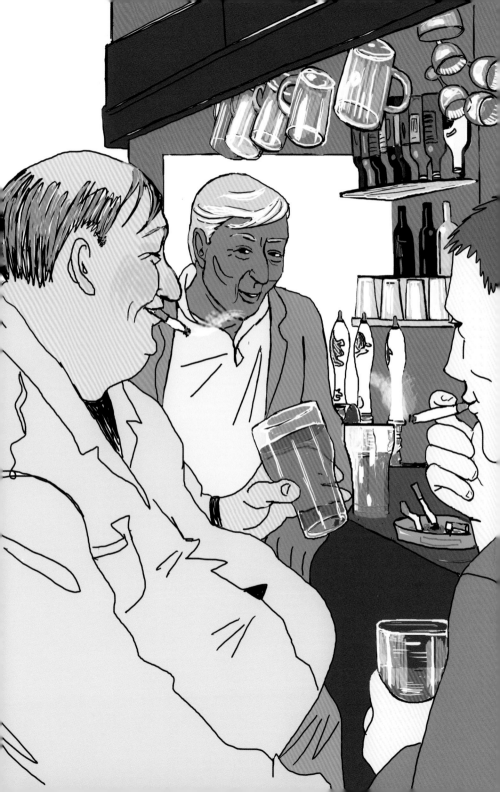

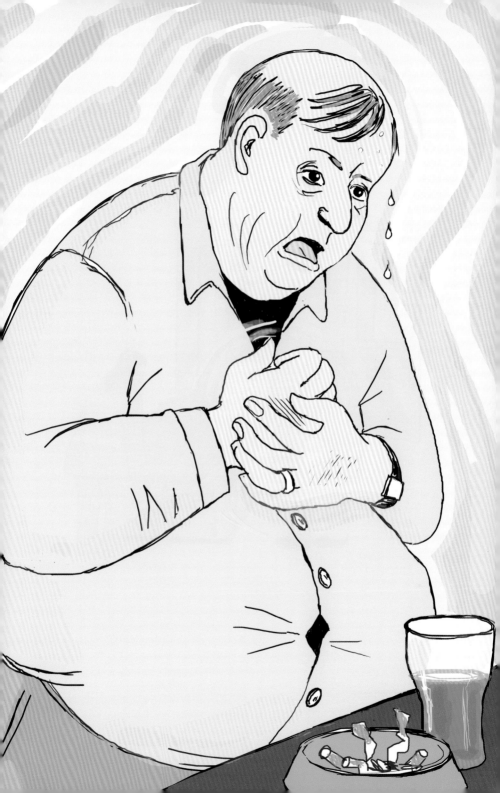

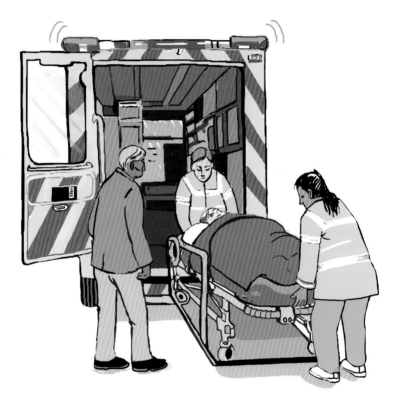

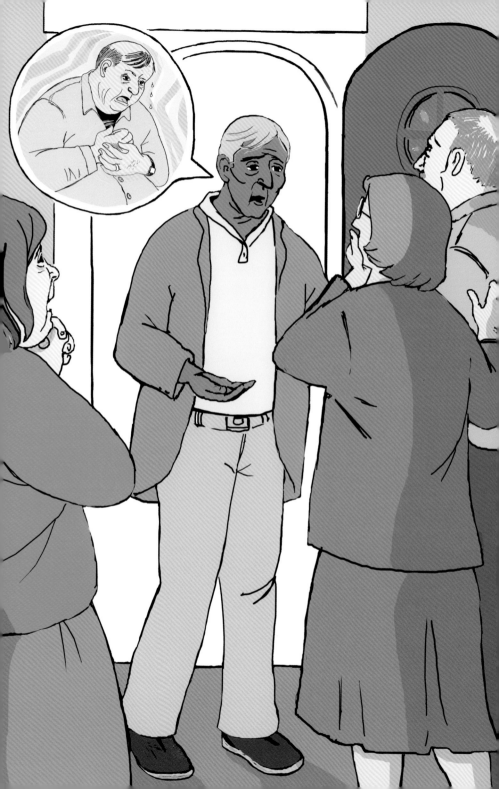

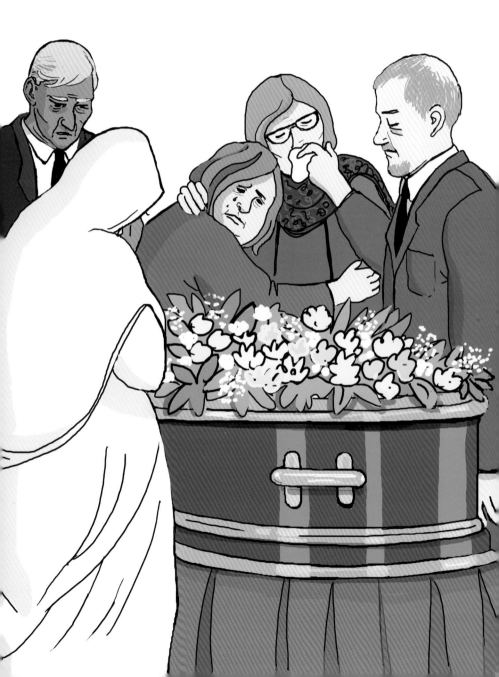

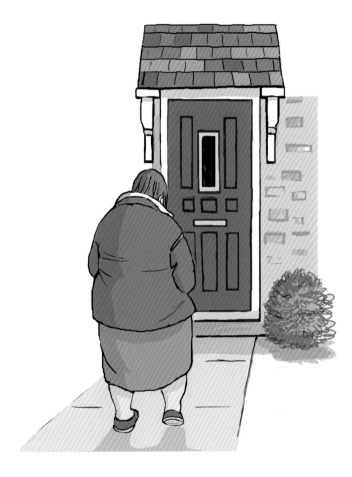

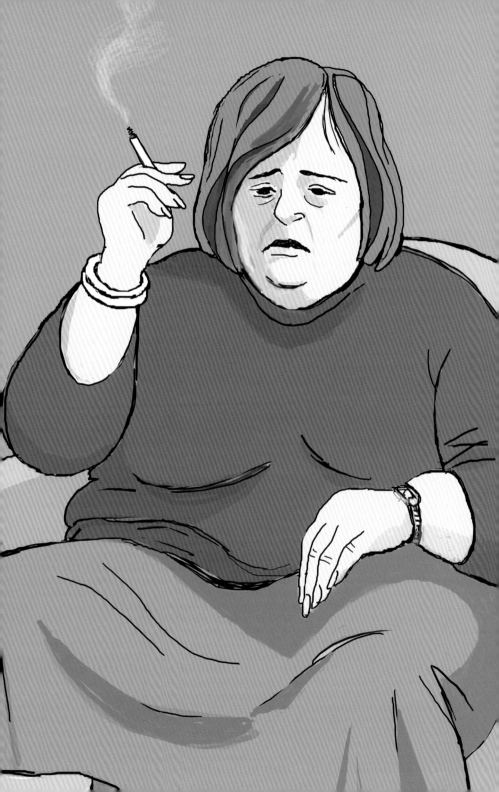

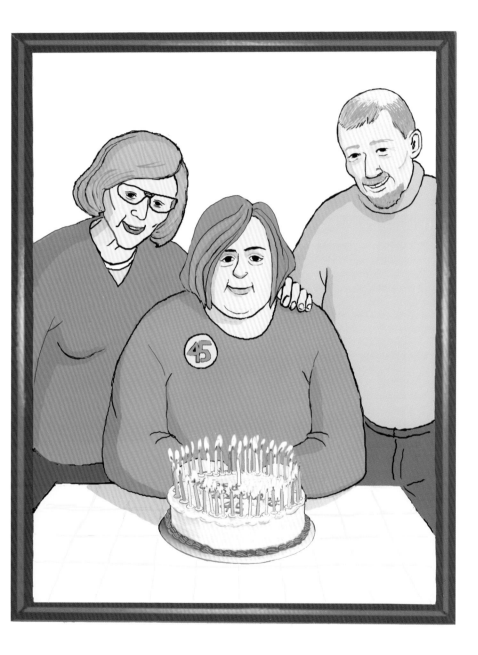

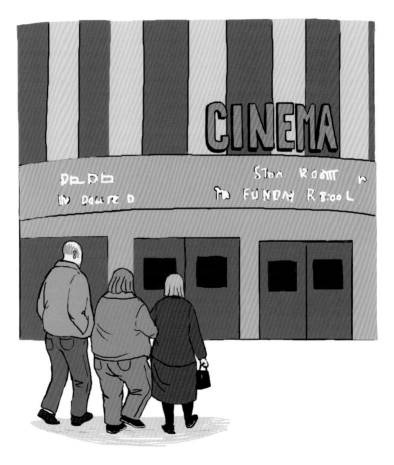

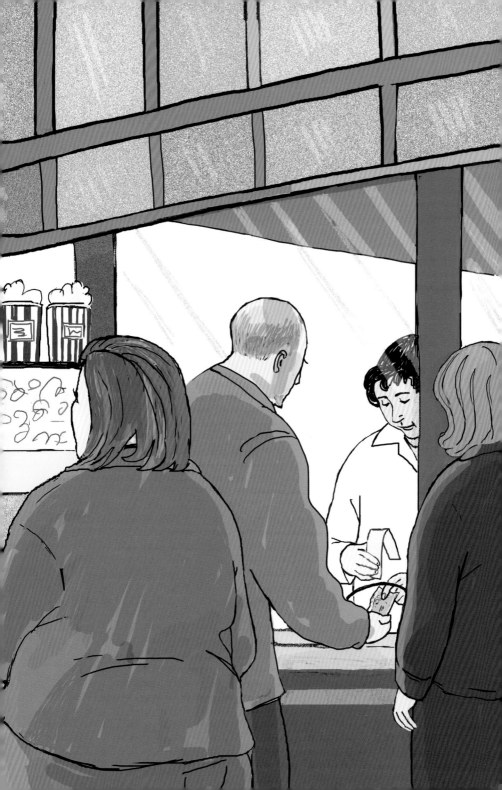

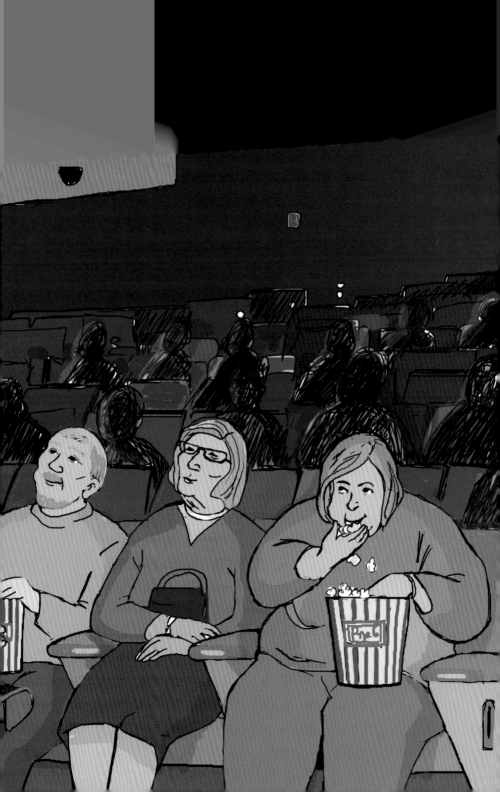

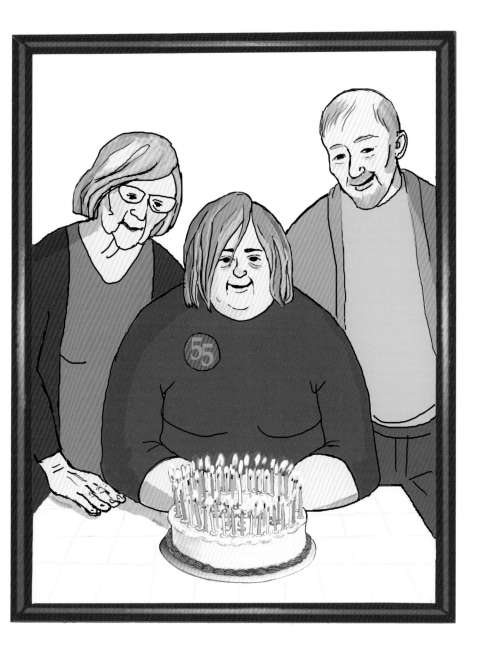

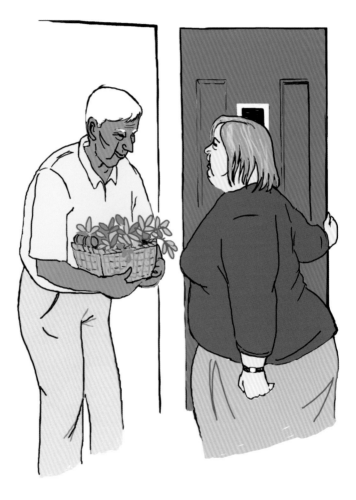

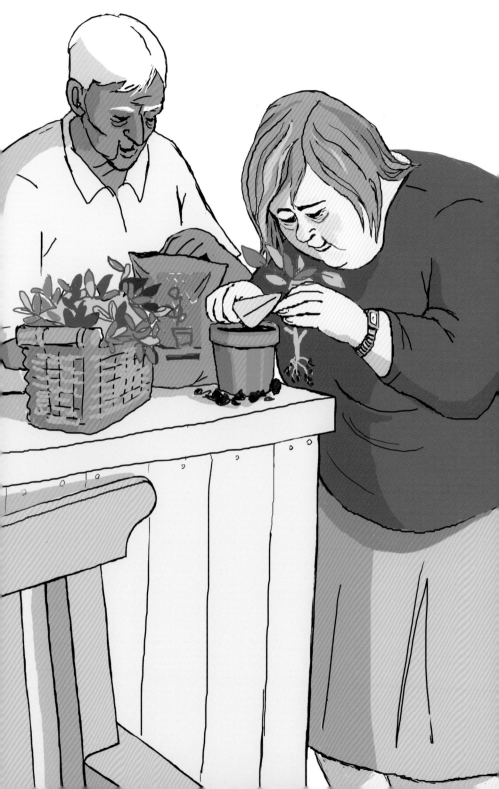

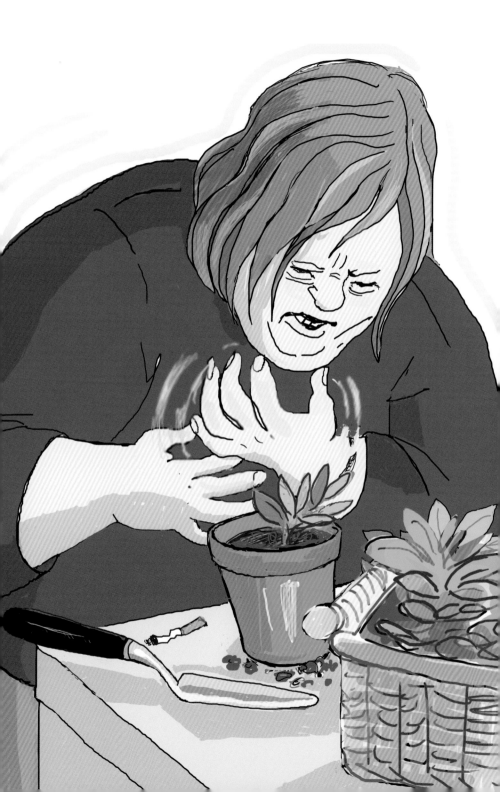

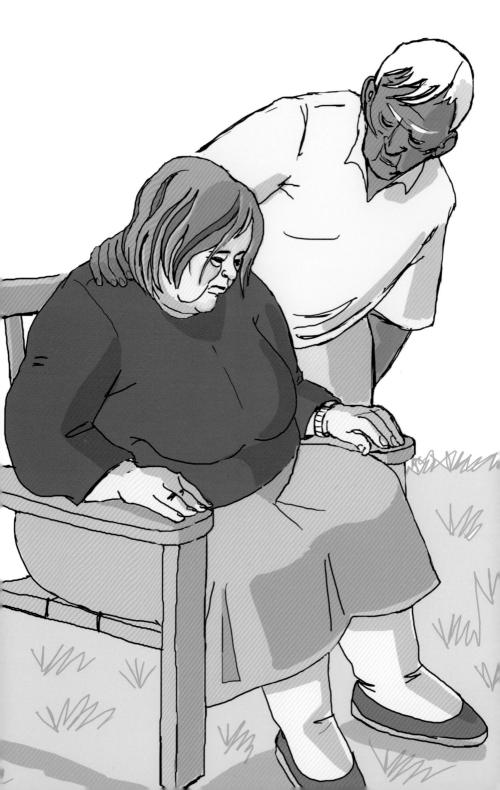

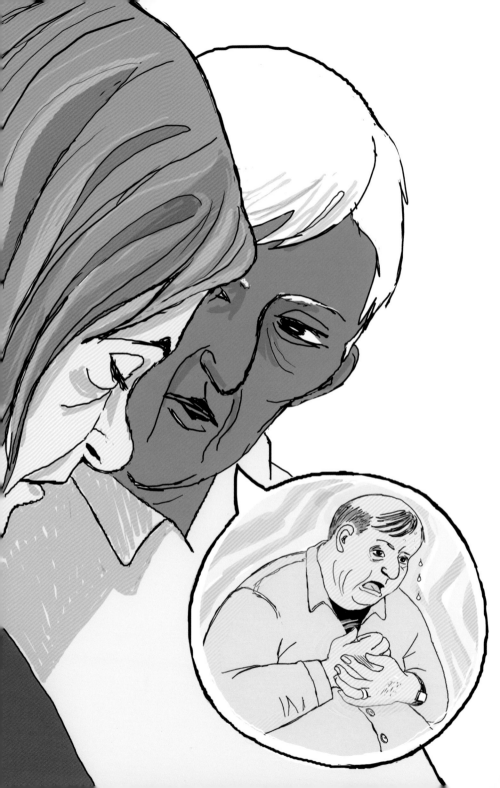

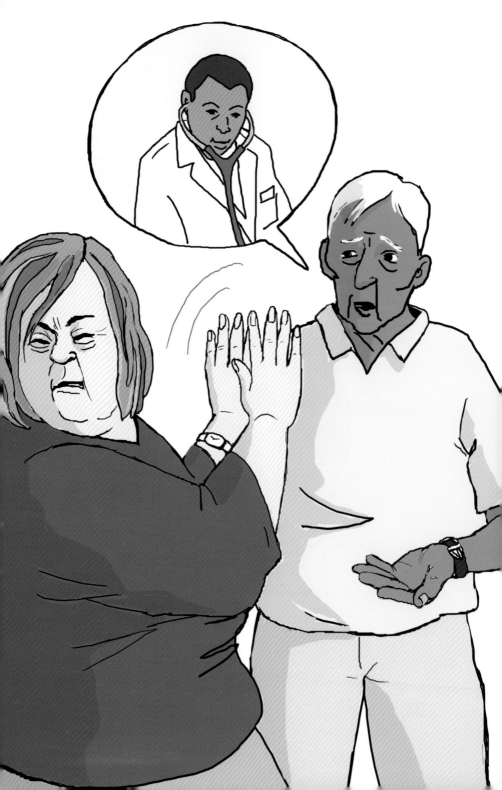

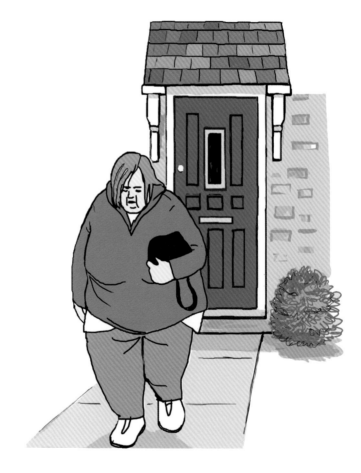

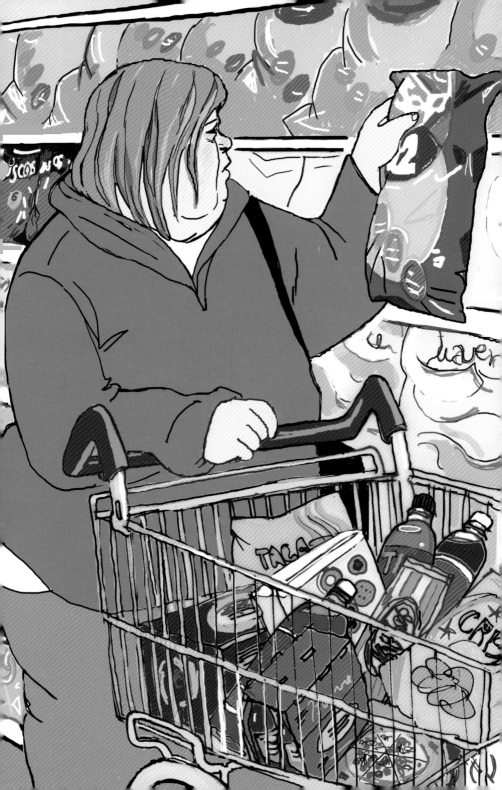

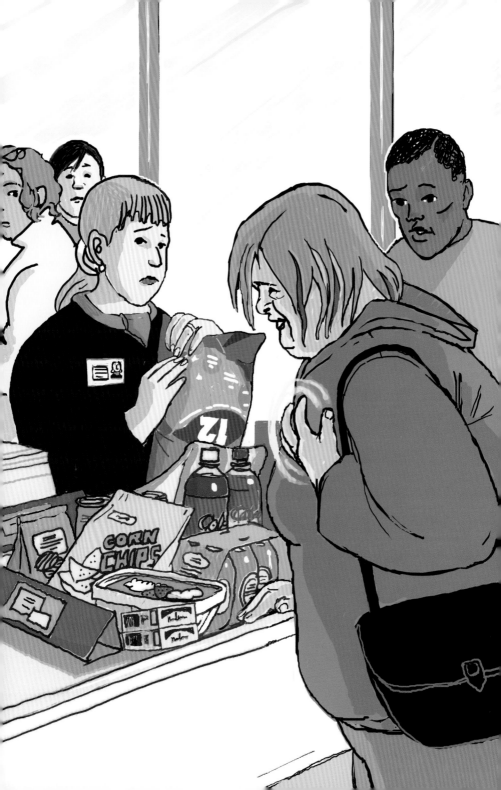

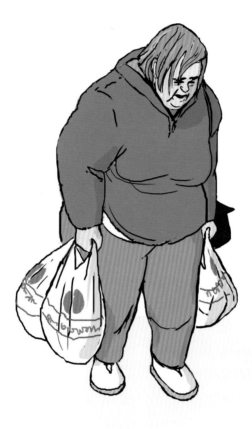

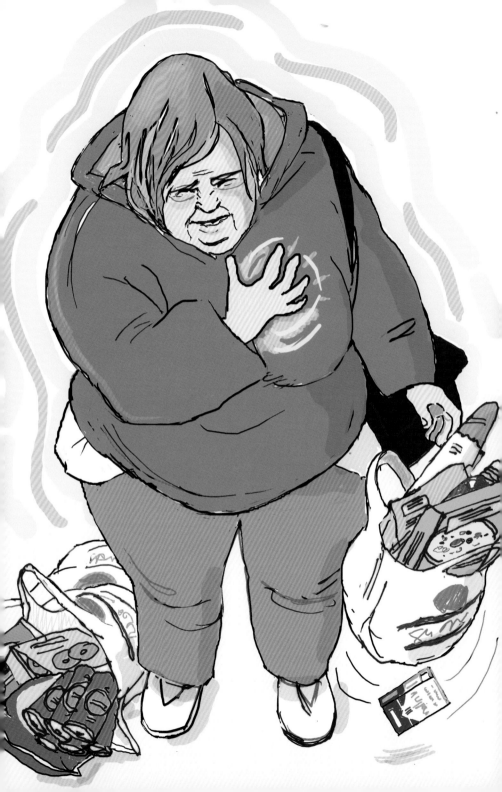

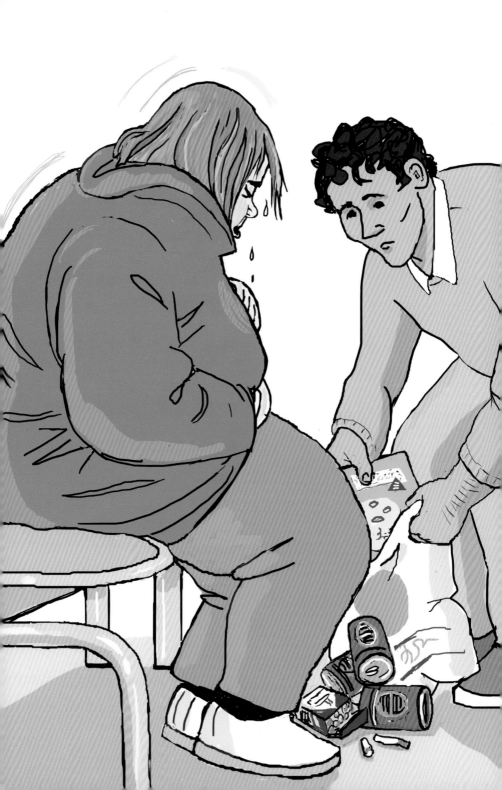

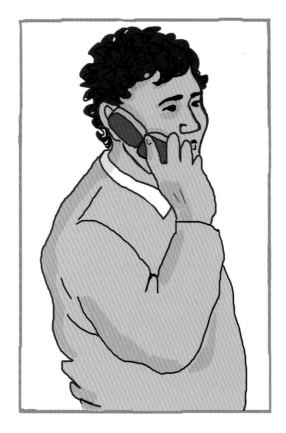

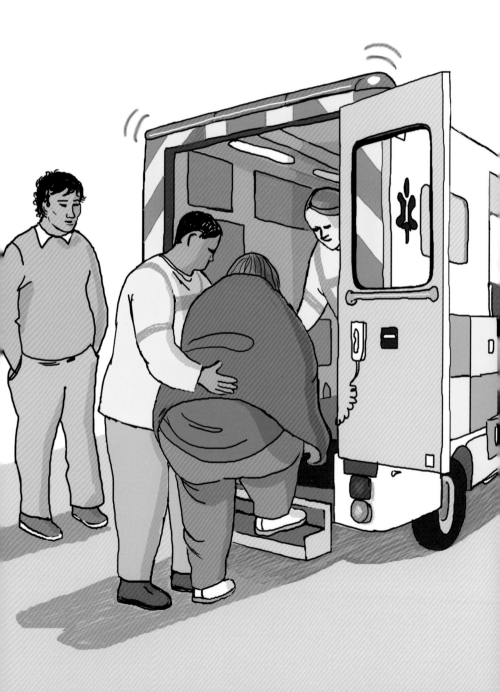

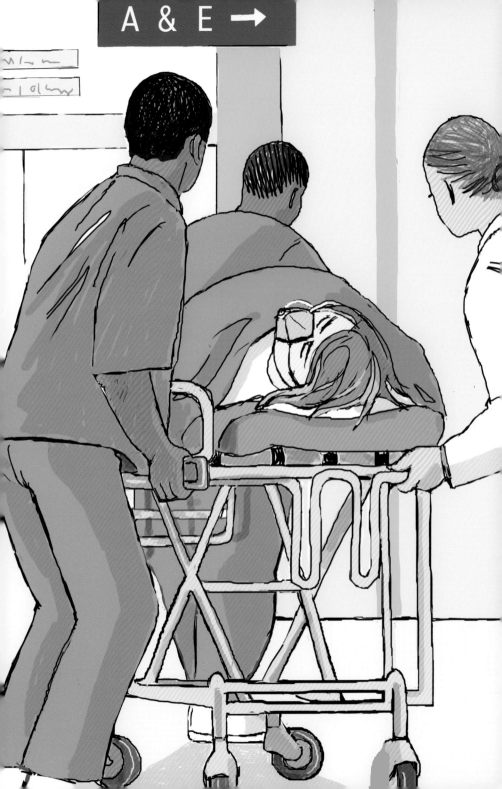

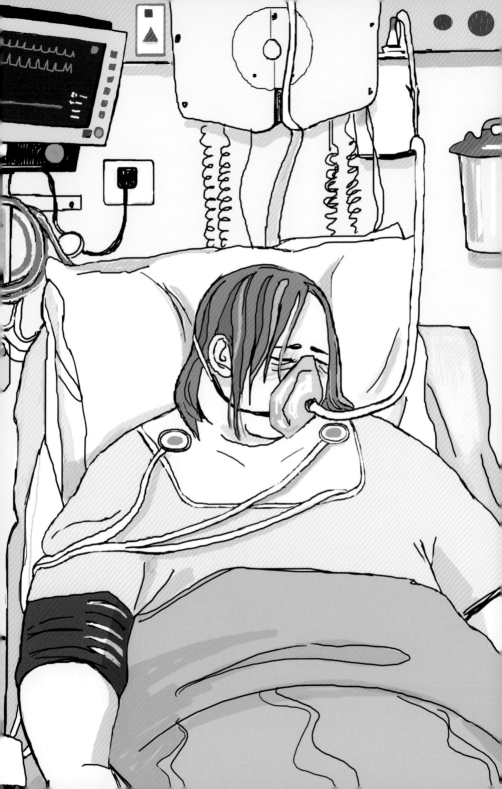

33

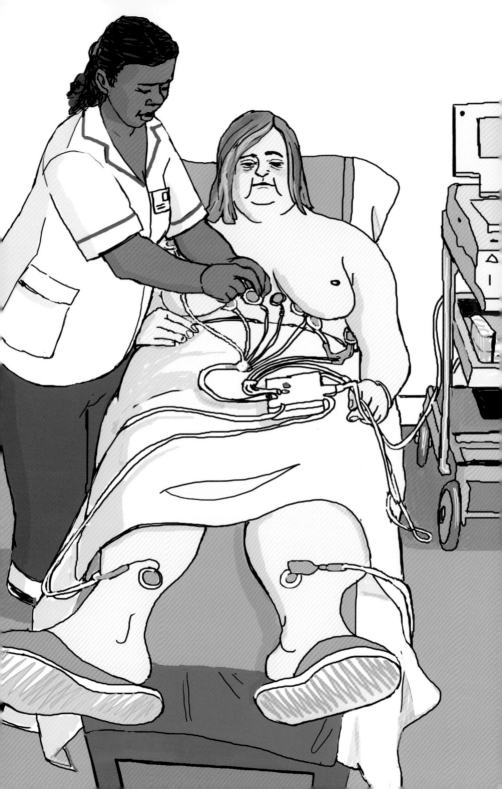

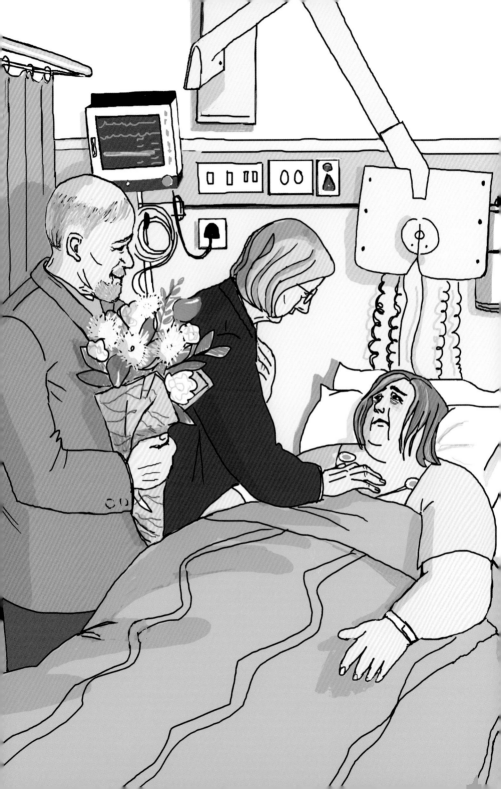

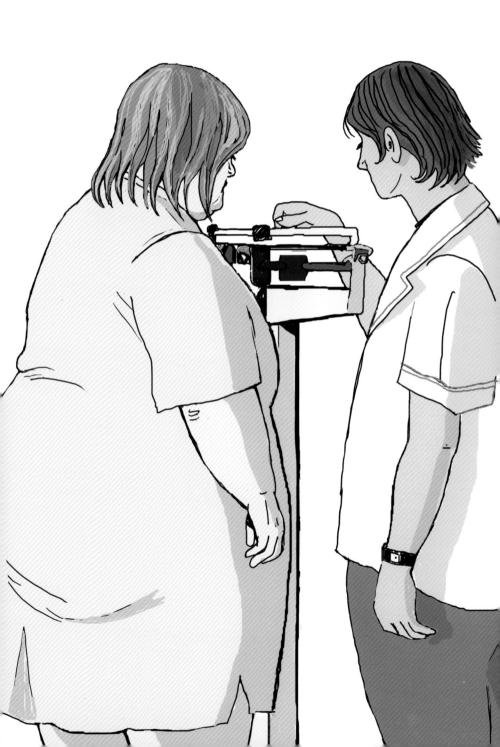

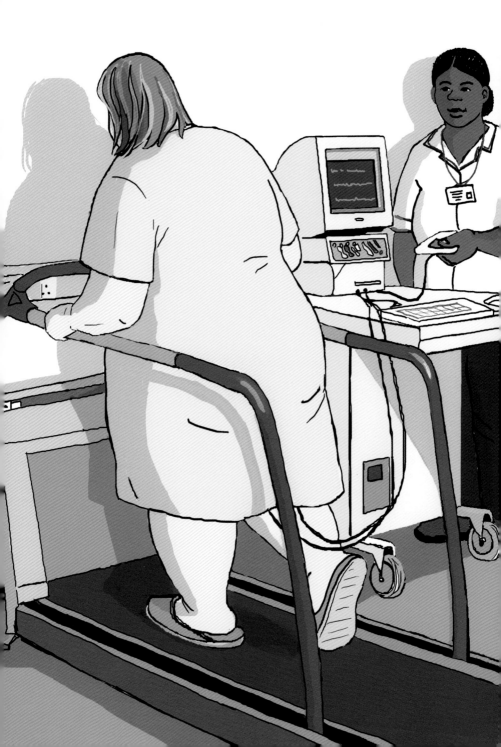

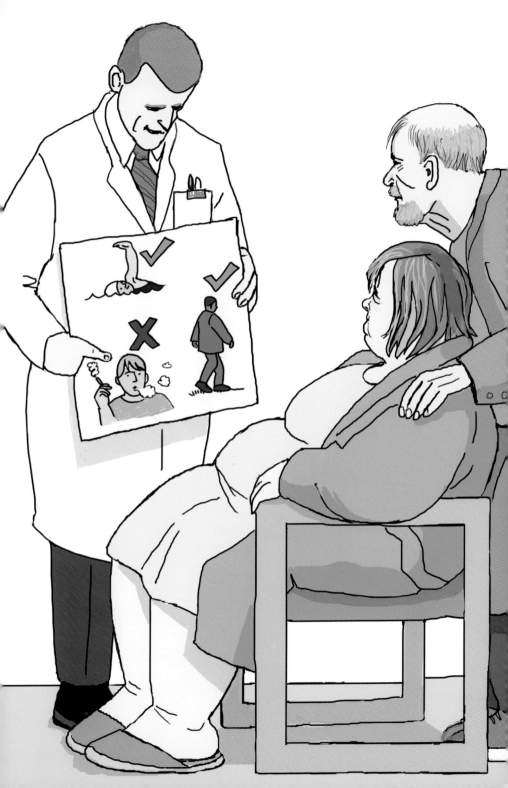

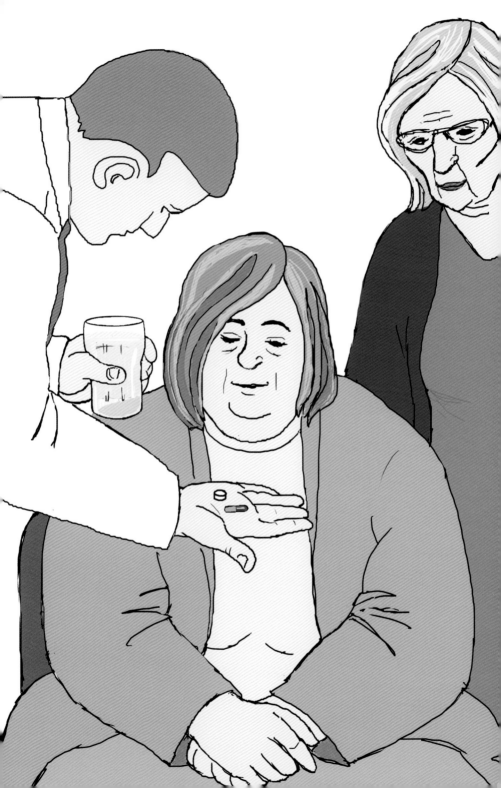

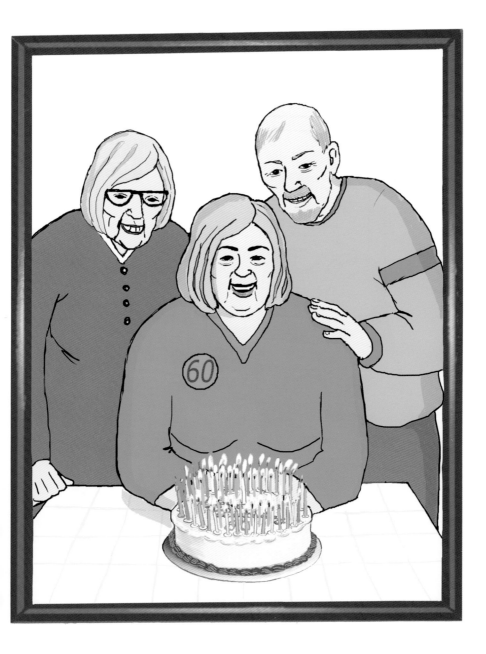

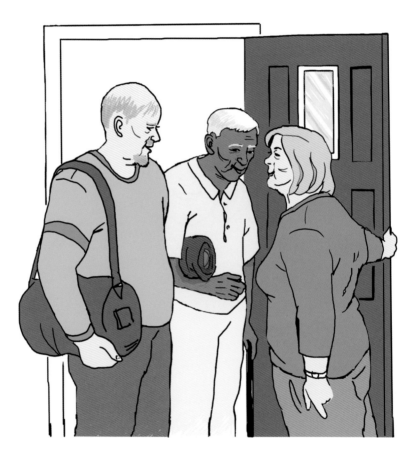

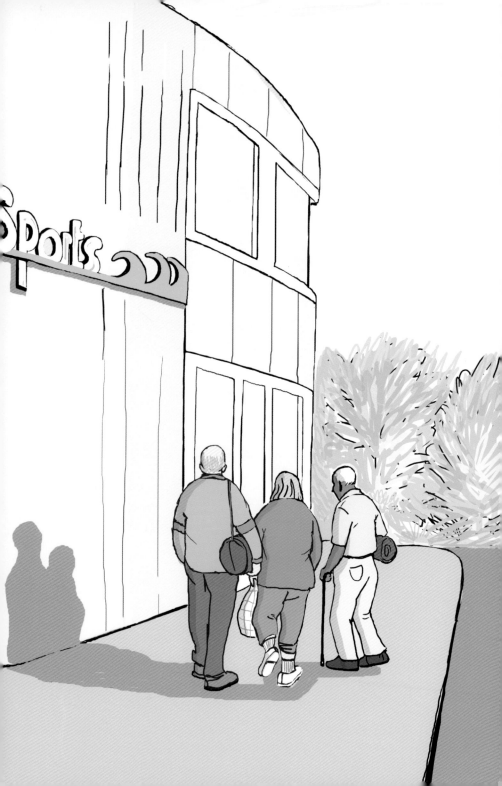

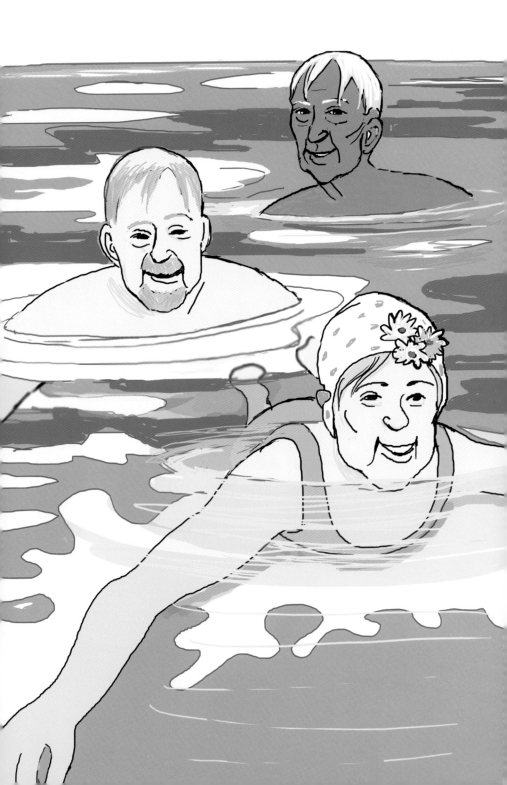

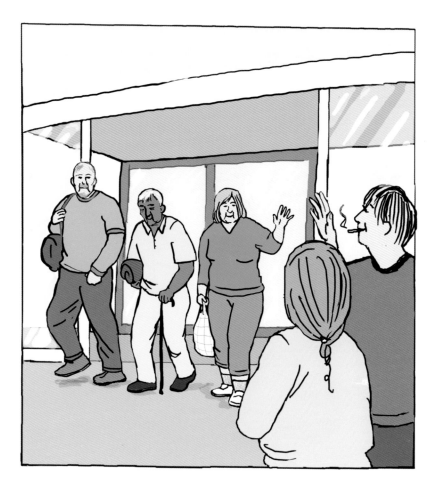

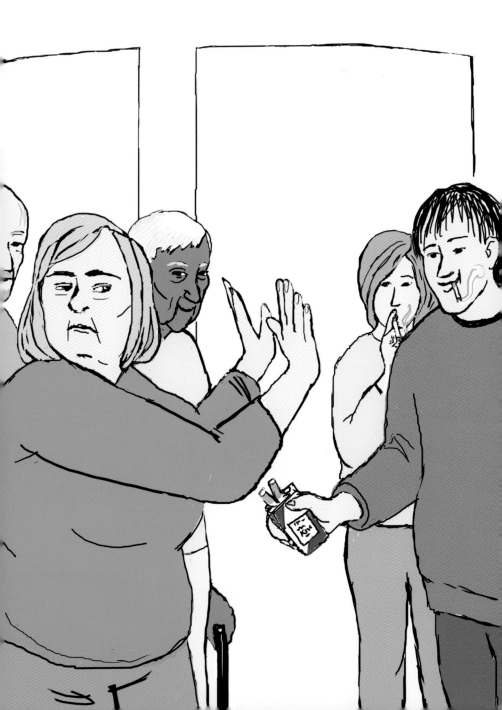

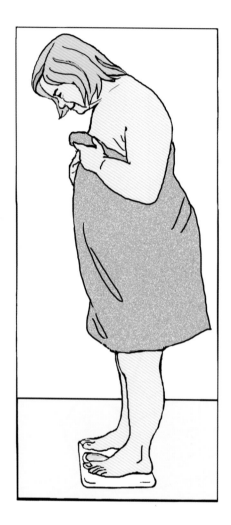

43

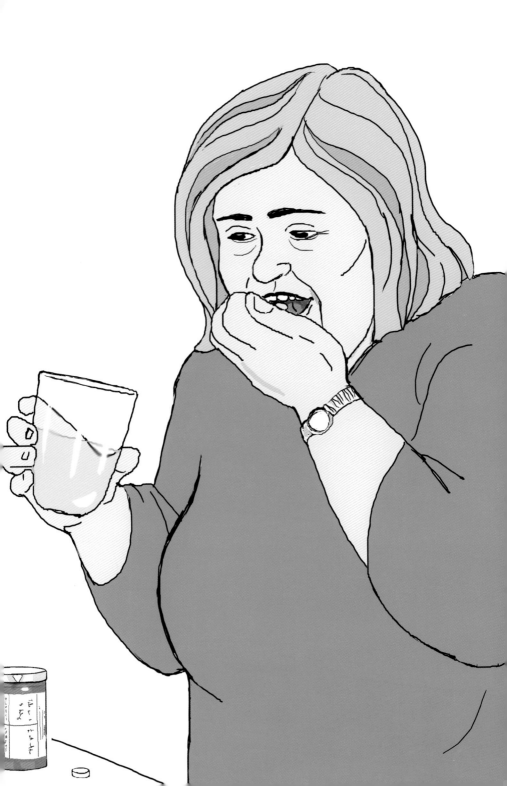

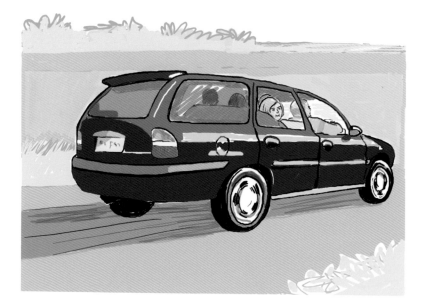

44

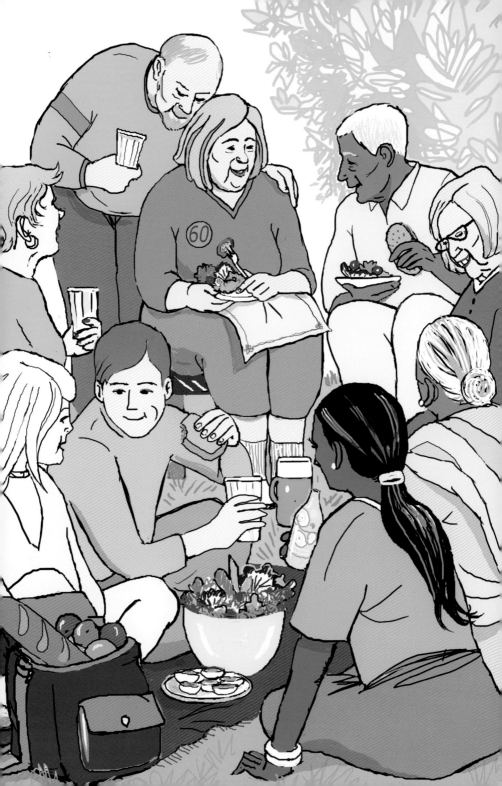

The following words are provided for people who want a ready-made story rather than tell their own

1. Jane is 25. She will celebrate her birthday with her father, mother and brother.

2. Jane is getting ready for a party. She is 25 today.

3. She enjoys herself with her friends and family.

4. Jane says goodbye to her family and a friend.

5. Jane relaxes after the party. She smokes a cigarette and has a beer. She's looking at the mess.

6. Jane and her family. Now she is 40.

7. Jane's skirt is too tight. She's getting fat, and she's still smoking.

8. Jane goes out. She is waiting for a bus. Oh dear, she's smoking again.

9. It's party time again. Everyone has come to Jane's birthday.

10. Some people are dancing. Some are chatting. Jane is eating cake, but she doesn't look happy.

11. Her Dad goes to the pub with his friend Ali.

12. They have a drink and a chat in the pub.

13. Dad gets a bad pain in his chest.

14. An ambulance comes to take Dad to hospital. Dad's friend Ali goes to see Jane and her Mum and Jeff. He tells them that Dad has had a heart attack.

15. Dad dies. Everyone is very sad.

16. Jane misses her Dad.

17. Jane is 45. Here she is with her Mum and her brother.

18. Jane's Mum and brother take her to the cinema for a birthday treat.

19. They all like the film. Jane is eating lots of popcorn.

20. Now Jane is 55. Everyone in the family is getting older.

21. Her Dad's friend Ali helps her to do some gardening.

22. Then Jane has a bad pain in her chest.

23. Ali is worried about Jane. He helps her to sit down.

24. Ali reminds Jane about her father. He tells her about the pain her Dad had. He thinks she has the same kind of pain.

25. Jane doesn't want to go to see her doctor.

26. Jane gets on with her life. She goes shopping.

27. Jane has chest pain again. This time the pain comes on at the checkout.

28. She tries to carry her shopping home, but the pain comes back.

29. Another shopper helps Jane. He picks up her shopping and puts it back in her bags.

30. He phones for an ambulance. Jane gets into the ambulance.

31. The ambulance takes Jane to hospital. She feels dreadful. She has an oxygen mask on her face.

32. Jane is in bed on a ward. She is wired up to all sorts of things. She's still got an oxygen mask on.

33. She's having a heart test. It's called an ECG.

34. Jane's brother and mother visit her in hospital.

35. Jane is on the scales. She is being weighed. She looks very heavy.

36. She's having another heart test. This time she has to walk on the treadmill at the same time.

37. The doctor tells Jane she can go swimming and walking. He tells her how to get fit.

38. The doctor tells Jane to take some pills.

39. Here is her family. Jane looks better now she's 60. She's looking after her health.

40. Jane works hard to get fit. She goes to the Sports Centre several times a week.

41. She loves swimming.

42. Jane says hello to her friends. One of them offers her a cigarette. She says "No!". Jane has stopped smoking. She is looking after her heart.

43. She watches her weight. And she remembers to take her pills.

44. Jane and her family go off to the country. She celebrates her 60th birthday with a picnic.

What is heart disease?

Heart disease or coronary heart disease (CHD) happens when your arteries become narrowed through a process called atherosclerosis. When this happens the blood and oxygen supply to the heart muscle is reduced, particularly when you exercise and the demands on the heart muscle increase.

The heart muscle needs oxygen to make it work, and it needs more oxygen when people do exercise. Oxygen gets into your blood when you breathe and the blood takes the oxygen to your heart. If the arteries are narrowed, then it's hard for the heart to get enough oxygen.

What are the symptoms of heart disease?

The main symptom of heart disease is chest pain. This is known medically as *angina*, caused by insufficient oxygen reaching your heart muscle. Angina is a feeling of heaviness, tightness or pain, usually in the middle of your chest. You may have pain in your arms, neck, jaw, face, back or stomach. It usually starts during exercise. For example, it may come on if you run for a bus, play a game such as tennis or football, climb stairs or walk uphill. It may come on in cold weather, after a heavy meal, or when you are feeling stressed. It can stop once you stop what you are doing, or when you take medication.

Unfortunately for many people the first sign that something is wrong is a heart attack. This is medically known as *myocardial infarction*, which happens when the blood supply to a part of the heart muscle stops altogether.

Usually a heart attack happens because of a blood clot in one of the arteries (known as coronary arteries). The pain of a heart attack may be very bad, or may be mistaken for indigestion, but unlike angina it does not go away. Other symptoms may include sweating, light-headedness, feeling sick or breathlessness. Unlike angina, these do not get better by resting.

How can you tell if someone is having a heart attack?

The following symptoms are sometimes due to coronary heart disease. They can be harmless or due to other medical conditions. If you, or someone you care for, ever experience any of them it is a good idea to see your doctor.

- Unusual breathlessness when doing light activity or at rest, or breathlessness that comes on suddenly.

- Angina – chest pain, heaviness or tightness in the chest that comes on during exertion or emotional stress, and that may spread to the arms, neck, jaw, face, back or stomach.

- Palpitations – awareness of your heartbeat or a feeling of having a fast and unusually forceful heartbeat, especially if it lasts for several hours or comes back over several days and causes chest pain, breathlessness or dizziness.

- Fainting – fainting can happen when your brain does not get enough oxygen. There are many reasons for fainting so you should ask your doctor about it. It is not always a serious symptom.

- Oedema – the medical word for fluid retention or puffiness caused by an abnormal build up of fluid in tissue such as ankles, legs, lungs and stomach.
- Cyanosis – the medical word for bluish fingernails or lips. It can be a result of too little oxygen in the blood.
- Fatigue or feeling tired is a very common symptom with many causes, including depression.
- **Severe crushing chest pain** may be a heart attack. It may come on when you are resting or after exercise, and be accompanied by
  - sweating
  - light-headedness
  - feeling sick
  - shortness of breath.

If this pain lasts for more than 15 minutes, dial 999 and ask for an ambulance.

The next page shows you **what to do** if someone has a heart attack and is unconscious. Do not attempt to resuscitate the person unless you have received training.

There are two parts to resuscitation. One is performing chest compressions (cardiopulmonary resuscitation – CPR) to try to get the heart working again. The second part is mouth-to-mouth resuscitation (artificial respiration).

First aid courses are offered all over the country at evening classes or by voluntary organisations such as St John Ambulance or the British Red Cross (see www.sja.org.uk and www.redcross.org.uk).

What to do if someone has a heart attack

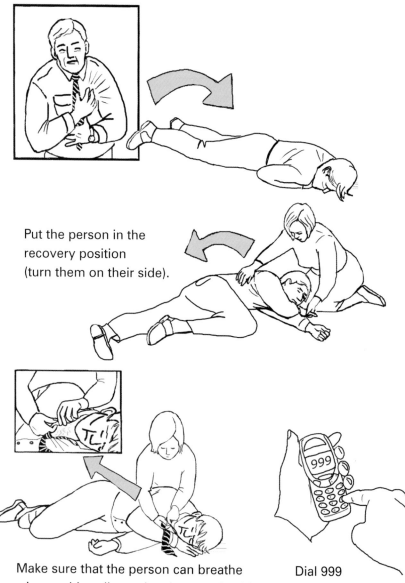

Put the person in the
recovery position
(turn them on their side).

Make sure that the person can breathe
– loosen his collar and make sure that his
airway is clear.

Dial 999
for an ambulance.

What causes heart disease?

Some causes of heart disease are well known, some are not. Some things make it more likely. These are known as risk factors. There are some risk factors you cannot do very much about, such as your age, your gender or your ethnic group. You may have some control over some other risk factors. For instance, you may be able to control what you eat, whether you smoke and the amount of exercise you take. It can be harder for people with learning disabilities to take control of their diet and exercise. This is because they may not understand how important each is. Or it may be because their carers don't know how important diet and exercise are. Often it's someone's carer who chooses their food and their daily activities. Sometimes the carer knows someone is eating the wrong food or taking insufficient exercise, but feels it is that person's choice. Sometimes thinking the person has 'the right to choose' may actually put a vulnerable person at risk and this means that families and other carers are actually failing to exercise a duty of care.

Risk factors

The most important risk factors for heart disease include:

- Your age – the risk of developing heart disease increases with age.
- Your gender – many people think of coronary heart disease as being a male problem. However, this is far from being the case. In fact coronary heart disease is responsible for more deaths of women than any

other disease. This risk becomes even greater after the change (the menopause).

- Your genes – if you have a family history of coronary heart disease, then you are more at risk of developing it yourself.

- Your ethnic background – if you are Black or south Asian you are more at risk of heart disease, although for different reasons. For instance, if you are south Asian you have a higher risk of developing diabetes, which is a risk factor for heart disease. If you are Black you are more at risk of high blood pressure, a separate risk factor for heart disease.

- Diabetes – diabetes is a disease which does not allow the body to clear the sugar that accumulates in the blood and this causes harm to the blood vessels. If you have diabetes you are three times more likely to develop coronary heart disease. Unfortunately, because in the early stages diabetes often has no symptoms, in many people diabetes remains undetected for years, during which time the arteries become more damaged.

- Being overweight and inactive – both of these are separate risk factors for heart disease, and also increase your risk of developing diabetes in middle age. It is important to be active. Exercise, like going to the gym regularly or having a half-hour walk every day, is very useful to protect the heart from coronary heart disease. The best level of exercise is what we call dynamic exercise, for example running, cycling, swimming and playing sports like tennis, badminton and squash. Less useful exercise is what we call isometric exercise, such as weightlifting.

- High blood pressure – the higher the blood pressure the higher the risk of heart disease. The main factors leading to high blood pressure are being over-weight, too much salt in what we eat and drink and inactivity.

- Raised cholesterol levels – cholesterol causes our arteries to become narrower. Cholesterol is in some of the fat that we eat (called saturated fat), but we also produce it in our body. The fat on meat, in butter and in oils like coconut and palm oil is saturated fat, and we can eat less of these. Or we can take medicine to reduce the cholesterol level in our blood.

- Alcohol – don't drink too much alcohol. A small amount of alcohol, like a glass of wine a day, can be good for your heart. Anything more than that can damage your heart. It is dangerous to drink a lot of alcohol on the same day – this is called binge drinking or getting drunk.

How is heart disease treated?

The treatment of heart disease varies depending on your age and how serious it is. Firstly we'll think about how to stop heart disease developing. To prevent heart disease the best thing you can do is to keep fit by taking physical exercise regularly, by not putting on weight and by having a healthy diet with:

- less saturated fat
- at least five portions of fruit and vegetables a day
- less salt
- a limited amount of sugar.

It is also important to stop smoking if you do, or never take up smoking.

If you have risk factors for heart disease it is important to control those, possibly with the use of drugs from your doctor. Blood pressure medications reduce high blood pressure. Tablets to lower cholesterol are used to control the levels of cholesterol in the blood, and tablets to control diabetes are also available.

Secondly, if you have developed heart disease there are a number of other medications you can take according to your symptoms, including blood-thinning drugs like aspirin, beta blockers or ACE inhibitors. Anti-arrhythmic drugs can be prescribed if your heart beats irregularly. All these will be decided by your doctor following a clinical examination. If you have had a heart attack you should have a programme of rehabilitation as soon as possible. This will help you to regain your energy and your ability to exercise.

Rehabilitation

Patients who have had a heart attack usually receive a cardiac rehabilitation programme. These start about 4 weeks after the heart attack, and involve going once or twice a week for between 6 and 12 weeks – or longer. The programme might be run at the local hospital or at a nearby health centre. Patients may also be able to follow a rehabilitation programme at home.

The aim of cardiac rehabilitation is to help recovery and restore as full a life as possible. Cardiac rehabilitation can benefit all patients, whether mildly or severely limited by heart disease. Those with mild heart disease may even find that following a rehabilitation programme makes them fitter than before.

Rehabilitation programmes vary throughout the country, but most programmes cover three areas:

- exercise
- relaxation
- information on lifestyle and treatment.

Where to find help and advice

American Heart Association   www.americanheart.org

The American Heart Association publishes an extremely wide range of books, fact sheets and leaflets and its website, though obviously geared for the USA, contains much useful and relevant information on prevention and self-help.

Action on Smoking and Health (ASH)

102 Clifton Street   Telephone: 020 7739 5902
London EC2A 4HW   www.ash.org.uk

ASH is a national campaigning charity with branches throughout the UK. It works at many levels to tackle problem of smoking and smoking-related diseases and their effects. It provides useful information on quitting or cutting down smoking.

British Heart Foundation (UK)

14 Fitzhardinge Street   Telephone: 020 7935 0185
London W1H 6DH   Information Line: 08450 70 80 70
                            www.bhf.org.uk

The British Heart Foundation is a charity working to fight against heart disease. It publishes a range of excellent leaflets on various aspects of heart disease. Its comprehensive website has a Healthy Heart section describing links between heart disease and smoking, alcohol, physical exercise, diet, stress and high blood pressure. It also funds and coordinates the Heartstart UK initiative, which promotes and develops emergency life support training throughout the UK.

Chest, Heart & Stroke Scotland

Head Office
65 North Castle Street
Edinburgh EH2 3LT

Advice line: 0845 077 6000
E-mail: adviceline@chss.org.uk
www.chss.org.uk

This organisation aims to improve the quality of life of people in Scotland affected by chest and heart illness, through medical research, advice and information, and support in the community.

HEART UK

7 North Road
Maidenhead
Berkshire SL6 1PE

Telephone: 01628 628 638
E-mail: ask@heartuk.org.uk
www.heartuk.org.uk

HEART UK is committed to raising awareness of heart disease in the UK and publishes a wide range of information sheets, dietary advice and newsletters for patients and families with inherited high cholesterol.

Heart Health Promotion Website

www.shef.ac.uk/uni/projects/mshhp

Sponsored by the Department of Health, this website provides easy-to-use information relating to heart health, and is aimed at young people. It gives information on heart disease as it affects different people, including Black and minority ethnic groups, and on nutrition, alcohol, smoking, exercise and substance misuse.

Patient UK

General: www.patient.co.uk
Coronary heart disease: www.patient.co.uk/
showdoc/26739411

A very informative website that provides leaflets and factsheets about health, including coronary heart disease, patient support and self-help. The information is easy to access, all medical and unfamiliar terms are explained and, where necessary, helpful diagrams are included.

Some other titles in the Books Beyond Words series

Using health services is explained in to *Going to the Doctor, Going to Out-Patients* and *Going into Hospital*. In *Getting on with Cancer* a woman has radiotherapy, chemotherapy and surgery. The book shows the unpleasant side of treatment, but ends on a positive note.

Looking After My Breasts and *Keeping Healthy 'Down Below'* are designed to support women who are invited for breast screening or for a smear test. Feelings, consent and health education are addressed in both books.

Looking After My Balls is designed to help men with learning disabilities to learn more about their testicles and about how to look after them.

Getting on with Epilepsy shows that it is possible to enjoy an active life with epilepsy, and illustrates activities such as safe drinking, swimming and cooking.

Food . . . Fun, Healthy and Safe includes do's and don'ts to prevent choking, general advice on eating well and outlines of special diets.

George Gets Smart is about personal cleanliness and shows how a man's life changes when he learns to keep clean and smart.

Susan's Growing Up shows how a young girl is helped to cope with her first menstruation by her teacher at school and by her mother.

To order copies (at £10.00 each; 10% reduction for 10 or more books) or for a leaflet giving more information, please contact: Book Sales, Royal College of Psychiatrists, 17 Belgrave Square, London SW1X 8PG. Credit card orders can be taken by telephone (020 7235 2351, extension 146).